Steps & Traditions for Dualaholics

Hints from a Sponsor

Study Edition for Anonymous Meetings of
Dual Diagnosed Alcoholic, Emotion, Narcotic
and Family Fellowships

Michael B.

© 2018, Michael B. Self-published unless and until Conference approved.

ISBN: 9781980522232

Imprint: Independently published

Nonfiction > Medical > Mental Health

Nonfiction > Self-Help > Twelve-Step Programs

To Jerry A.

Table of Contents

Mike's Story 1
Step One 9
Step Two 13
Step Three 17
Step Four 21
Step Five 24
Step Six 26
Step Seven 28
Step Eight 31
Step Nine 33
Step Ten 35
Step Eleven 37
Step Twelve 39
The Traditions 43
    Tradition One 43
    Tradition Two 43
    Tradition Three 43
    Tradition Four 44
    Tradition Five 44
    Tradition Six 45
    Tradition Seven 45
    Tradition Eight 46
    Tradition Nine 46
    Tradition Ten 47
    Tradition Eleven 47
    Tradition Twelve 48

Mike's Story

As this is a personal story, I am going to take the liberty of using the personal first-person pronoun. In the rest of the book, I will write as if for the community of Dualaholics, so the collective pronoun we will be used. Of course, that may be taking a greater liberty. That is up for the reader to decide.

When I was eight and living with my family at My grandmother's house, my cousin who was eighteen was legal and got to have a beer after lunch. I was jealous. A few years later, we had moved to a little town called Enon, Ohio. That summer, my father let me taste his beer. It tasted like it's name and I was not impressed.

The next summer, we moved around the block and after exploring the lot behind our house, I came in and took a deep gulp of what I thought was a glass of water. It was my mother's martini, which they immediately took away from me. Too late. It went to my head and I had found a new God.

Around the same time, I found a government book in the village library. I thought that the chart showing the organization of the government looked messy with too many independent agencies.

I felt the agencies should have been assigned to departments, and that some of the departments should be combined, creating a Department of Science. (I still think so, but now I have a government degree.) Later, when I found out that President Carter had reorganized his state government that way, I thought that I should be on his staff at the age of 16.

I also thought I could cure cancer and invent a water powers car (or rather, a hydrogen powered one that used power from the alternator to separate the water molecules). It should also be a hover craft. You can see where I am going with this.

Because I am actually very smart, especially in the social sciences, I thought I could not go wrong. No one realized at the time that my problem was more than a good imagination, although my government teacher in high school thought it a bit strange when I showed her my chart showing how the government should be organized, but no intervention occurred.

I kept up the project. In college, I used the school mainframe as a word processor to lay out my agency by agency plan to reorganize the government based on their functions. That it was on computer paper made it look impressive. I sent copies to various congressional committees and my Senators. One wrote me a nice note on the bottom of the form letter and the other gave me an internship the next term. Except for a year back in Ohio when I was a Presidential Management Intern, I have not left the DC area since.

I drank like a gentleman through high school, meaning my father would let me have a beer or champagne once in a while if I behaved. Once, when I was in high school, I joined the neighborhood men in collecting picnic tables for the community pool Memorial Day Party. They gave me a few beers and I both caught a decent buzz and felt like I belonged.

Sporadic use continued until college. My first night at school I was bored and there was nothing on TV. Someone said there was a party down the hill and I was soon standing next to the keg. An upper Glassman remarked "Hey, I'm happy." I was happy too.

During my academic career and after, I did the NASA Space Station Bibliographic Index, did research for another bibliography on public administration, participated in the conceptual design for the factory of the future, and did multiple cost analyses for strategic nuclear weapons and operational costs.

Over seventeen years of drinking, I went to class or work still drunk from the night before. I reacted with anger when I read in my agency daily newsletter that there was a noontime meeting available. (That should be a screening question for intervention.)

I cured countless hangovers with asthma and blood pressure medication. I misused my government credit card on nightly drinking, paying the bill and using it again to keep drinking.

I almost earned a Darwin Award riding in a shopping cart down a hill toward a train trestle while visiting a friend . n New Jersey. By some miracle, he caught up to me.

I found hashish and magic mushrooms. I tried blow but did not like the high. It only kept me awake. The bipolar already put me up. I drank to come down. I drove drunk for my year back in Ohio. Back in D.C., because alcohol was my God, I sold the car to my father in Iowa rather than having a judge sentence me to A.A.

Back in Iowa for Christmas in 1997, I got stopped for drunken walking and was delivered to my family, who began planning an intervention for the following Christmas. I got sober in 1998 before they could.

My first attempt in 1987 does not count because I was doing it for fiancé and would leave meetings before the end of the Preamble. When I finally was done, I could not get a buzz and could not stay sober.

The day after my last drinks (two pitchers of Stout and a last snifter of Grand Mariner, which tasted like orange syrup), I loaded up on coffee, soda and sugar. Naturally, I had a wicked panic attack. I was watching an MTV pre-awards show special. They played the first few moments of every song ever featured on all the prior shows. This would freak anyone out.

I fled to the throne room to God to escape. I remembered what a friend told me, that I could teach many people or could die drunk. I took a shower and prayed to God to take the drink away. I offered the sacrifice of my last two fingers of bourbon, which went down the drain rather then down the hatch. The desire to drink was removed.

As I had been engaged to a bipolar alcoholic, so I knew that I was entitled to chemical help. I called my HMO. They said to go to the Emergency Room. I did not trust them, thinking that you had to have your doctor refer you first to avoid a hefty bill. (I was mistaken).

I called my M.D. and the covering doctor gave me a scrip for a benzo. I had forgotten that I had a friend who could get me anything and that I already had a muscle relaxant that I could have detoxed on previously. Luckily, God gave me the gift of stupidity, which eventually got me to the rooms.

That was my first sobriety date, but later I changed it to when I was off meds. Later, be caused I have had to take the same meds for a mental health crisis and a heart attack in sobriety, I now celebrate on the original date, September 5th.

After the first scrip ran out, after stretching it for a week and not calling my doctor, I had another panic attack, this time from ruminating on how Star Trek, Deep Space Nine had ended, so I called the doctor for more. A different on-call doc gave me a few more pills and made me promise to call my own doctor during the week to get seen. He gave me nothing and told me I needed to call the HMO line again. I waited until after 5 and asked again. He said no, call them tomorrow and try and take a walk. I was in enough pain to finally listen, so I did.

When I was almost home, I thought if my father, who had passed three months before and began to cry. I had covered the pain by using, even smoking a spliff with my little brother the night before the funeral. It made me numb the next day, so I could not cry.

The next day, with low blood sugar, I set to work. I was in a fog about what to eat. Was sugar good or bad? Should I avoid fats? My mind was gone, but at least I got an OJ, which helped. I was in bad detox and could not work, so I went doctor shopping.

I called the health plan to get set up with a shrink and for talk therapy. The first doctor said no and I left a message with the second. I felt the need to go to the noon Mass nearby and fretted on the way how I could ever confess all my sins to my punishing God. At the exact time Mass was starting, Doc 2 called to leave a message. Miracle? I think so.

I tagged back and when I was on the phone to get the visits for talk therapy approved, she called back. No drugs until she could see me, so I switched back to the other line and asked for help. They sent me to a rehab a few blocks from home to get evaluated. I told my boss I would be out for a few days for mental health reasons.

On the subway to the hospital, I was beginning to freak out again when God put a friend on the train, who I went over to talk to. It held me together. When I got there, they asked me if I was suicidal. I said no, but the night was young. A hint: always say something like that if you need a bed.

The HMO gave me two days. I had missed dinner but they had ordered me a tray. I was overjoyed when it included green beans. The only vegetable I had gotten for weeks was the slaw you get with ribs when eating at the bar. Normalcy and more pills had arrived. They got me to an N.A. meeting, where I related in, sharing about getting high after my father's wake. Rehab sent me to aftercare, which got me to A.A. My rehab team never asked me anything about wanting to take over the planet and I did not tell them, so my bipolar disorder remained undiagnosed.

I had read about recovery supplements, which included Amino Acids that soothed the mind, and ordered them. A week out of rehab my feelings of despair returned. I called my counselor, who told me recovery hurts, I was feeling self-pity and to make a Gratitude List. The list worked, and the vitamins helped. I soon felt at home in Alcoholics Anonymous and launched into the Twelve Steps.

When I did my Fourth Step, the number of political and religious figures on my list had me think that I might be bipolar and that I would be told to leave A.A. and seek medical help. Rereading the Third Step in the *Big Book*, I identified with the politician who thought all would be Utopia if only people behaved.

This was enough for me to finish this step and go to the Fifth. My sponsor started me with my biggest secret (that I am the prophesied Prince Michael from Daniel, possibly the Archangel). He said that if you aren't filling this role today, it was not something to worry about today. He suggested that I share my delusion in a meeting. I found other saints and demons, many probably dualaholics. My worry about such issues pretty much evaporated. Oops.

A week later, I finished my eighth step list, banishing the politicians to people I would pray for and only a few days of prayer cured me of the need to do so. Six years later, I got into A.A. Service as a GSR, was on the track to Delegate but got sick with an adrenal tumor, knocking me off the track.

My service enhanced my recovery and hurt it as well. I had only service sponsees, which is not recommended. During this period, It I was diagnosed with adrenal disease and the meds during diagnosis wiped me out. I found out years later that I had probably had the tumor from the days when I was first reorganizing the government, et al, as such tumors can trigger hypomania, as well as high blood pressure and alcoholism. I was always doomed.

The tumor was removed and depression was a side effect, so it was back to the Vitamins, which helped, although too much 5HTP had me run for President in Americans Elect (see Step 12 on grandiosity). I shared this in meetings and this always got a laugh, but I was serious. My marriage and my life were falling apart. Budget sequestration cost me my job and my illness hurt my ability to work professionally. I was not honest with myself or practicing these principles in all my affairs.

During this time, my mother passed and my position as PTA president had me fully cooked. On a normal Sunday I was ruminating about the fact that I had gone through college so fast that I missed having a full experience. The self pity drove me over the edge into despair and I yelled at my daughter to stay away because I was feeling odd. I called my sponsor, who sent me to the E.R., leading to a psychiatric referral the next day.

This time, I got a full week of hospitalization. I brought A.A. literature, especially a stack of A.A. Grapevines, which I left there. I was feeling better but did not adequately share that I was having panic attacks while eating. It only got worse after discharge leading me to more E.R. visits and tranquilizers, which I took reluctantly. It took a while to figure out that antipsychotics don't work for me, even when they do, I need more tranquilizers.

Early therapy had me unearth emotions I thought were dealt with and two sponsors and several A.A. friends helped talk me down by phone on and after the bus ride home. After a change of doctors. I was off the anti-psychotics and the benzos. My wife saw a piece on *60 Minutes* about people who have almost total recall of past events, which is a form of Obsessive Compulsive Disorder. I tried an OCD med. It knocked me on my butt so thoroughly that I could not get off the couch.

I relied on a friend to get to meetings with a ride, but a walk to the store down the street was almost impossible. After the noon meeting and lunch, I was back on the couch in time for my wife to be disgusted with the slug I had become. Still these meetings and lunches were vitally important, as were finding sponsees. My brain and body were not working right, but my spirit was due to Alcoholics Anonymous.

A temp job and a theater job helped me stay married and get back into some kind of shape, but once we shifted from Chapter 13 bankruptcy to Chapter 7, I was on my own, staying in my old apartment with long commute to the theater each way. Soon, I lost the job and applied for Medicaid. I got a community health doctor and another anti-psychotic. These drugs do help many people, they just do not sit well with me. We all react to meds differently.

No money had me move into my sister's guest room (my stuff was already filling her garage). She helped me into a Psychiatric Rehabilitation Program and helped me try to find shelter, with no luck until someone in a meeting referred me to the Oxford Outreach Coordinator, who I met at a new house and became the first to open it (with almost 17 years, I was finally in a sober house). A.A. and my sister save my life again.

Soon, the new anti-psychotic started more panic attacks, which were really akathisia all along. The SSRI that had been working was expensive, so no one would put me back on it. Instead, I was on a different dopamine reuptake inhibitor and was OK until the following summer, when I finally got mental health housing (disability had come a few months earlier).

The dosage went down, but the symptoms persisted and I found a Dual Diagnosis meeting. The fellowship helped more than the content, as the meeting used a Step Guide from a prominent Midwestern rehabilitation hospital. It is written by therapists for alcoholics with mental illness and is more therapeutic than spiritual. It seemed like weak tea.

I wanted something by a fellow sufferer; another Dualaholic Dualist sounds like a western gunfighter movie and Dualic sings a little, but Dualaholic sings loud). The text just did not seem to "get it" as far as character flaws and God. My hope is that this text makes up for these lacks while still dealing with the special needs we all face.

Medicine changes were not easy and using a calcium channel blocker to step down the benzo had limited success. A try on an Gabapentin landed me in the hospital with a heart attack. The Gaba and Hydroxyzine that had helped me for years to sleep was withdrawn, the last for safety's sake. Back to the benzos. Eventually, after a month of insomnia and a doctor change, I was off the benzo, back on the hydro and sleeping. I did not adjust my sobriety date. That would have been false humility.

Part of the insomnia was due to a cyst on my throat, which stopped my breathing if I tucked my chin. The cyst and my beard had to go. It went and on day two after surgery, the only pain not due to intubation occurred when the drainage tube was removed and the stitches tightened.

On the train ride home, the pain was gone and I felt that peaceful easy feeling of opiates. This had me get of the train and go a meeting, where I and flushed the next pill down the Club's toilet. I never used another opiate. Part of that was hearing the stories of others who took the pain pills for too long and got addicted. While no one in bad pain should forsake necessary meds, getting off soon is always good.

It has been a few years since then my last crisis and my throat surgery. I am thriving. I have switched mood stabilizers and am of antipsychotics, which make me psychotic, and now take an antidepressant. I am also back in service below the group level as a General Service Representative.

It has been a year since I originally published this book. People seem to like it when I give them a copy. Maybe one day it will sell. That is in God's hands. Writing the book has been good for my recovery. If you find some benefit, it is icing on the cake.

In this text, I try to bring a bit more spirituality to the dual diagnosis literature. While I use some of the medical understanding I have picked up over the years, I will try to focus on the spiritual angle that books written by therapists cannot hope to reach. In the end, dualaholics, like alcoholics, find a spiritual awakening from one dualcoholic helping another.

I do not soft pedal character defects or God, which is often the flaw in literature created for us from outside the fellowship but I will present the need to find perfection in a very different light than Oxford, Dr. Bob and Bill W. presented it. I hope you find it helpful.

The suggested Traditions address the vital question of whether we should all continue in our respective fellowships or, to honor the Fifth Tradition, create a fellowship of our own. I hope this is use in our trudge to wellness.

In the text, I refer to the *Big Book* and the *Twelve & Twelve*, so chapters are much shorter than otherwise. This should help them be useful for reading in meetings.

Step One

*We admitted we were powerless over alcohol - that
our lives had become unmanageable.*

Sometimes, when you hit bottom, it is your idea. Often it is not, although to be willing to either work this program or work with your medical team on your mental health, you have to be honest with yourself about needing help. If you think you are not ready for either, then you aren't and more fun and pain awaits, both for you and your loved ones (for whom it won't be fun).

There are many ways to both reach the first step on alcohol and drugs and to finally be honest about the state of one's mind. There are also many theories about whether people become alcoholic and mentally ill or are born that way. The truth is that both are possible. There are, of course, three common ways to know you are Dualaholic.

A common way is to be diagnosed with a behavioral condition early in life, possibly after starting with attention deficit issues, depression, suicidal behavior or schizophrenia. Often, these young people were diagnosed before they could do much, if any, drinking and for a time, maintained compliance with directions to not mix their meds with alcohol. It is only later that alcohol is tried, and if there are no immediate consequences, tried with gusto. Some drugs, like benzos, when combined with alcohol, can make one an alcoholic. Other Dualaholics were genetically programmed and, once exposed, were doomed to recovery, hospitalizations, jails or death. These newcomers were used to a medical model for their recovery. It is only later that surrender to a spiritual program was necessary.

Another way to be diagnosed is to have a mental health crisis, such as a suicide attempt, hallucinations, a manic episode or other crisis where alcoholism is clearly present. This offers many opportunities for denial. Likewise, these people have to deal with two kinds of recovery at once, getting meds straight, learning about mental illness, finding a higher power and a spiritual program. The temptation to ignore one or the other disease is strong, but it could prove fatal. It is very possible, as "many of us do recover if we have the capacity to be honest."

Symptoms could have come separately or together. Some people can manifest bipolar disorder and drink at an early age, some may wait until late high school, college or early in their careers. Others may start drinking first, which may mask behavioral health symptoms. As strange as it sounds to some alcoholics, some never drink until much later than their original symptoms manifested, but were ignored. There are patterns, but no set rules.

When behavioral health symptoms are not strongly manifested but alcoholism is, doctors may not initially diagnose anything but alcoholism. The grandiosity of Bipolar II and of Alcoholism are not dissimilar. Sometimes, simple depression is diagnosed, an SSRI is given for a limited time and discontinued. For some, that is valid symptom management, but for others it could mask bigger problems. Alcoholics of this type may feel out of place in A.A. because they fear there is more wrong with them than the spiritual program can fix. They are likely to be right and the program does help, but not enough. This is another area where a great deal of honesty is required to seek additional help.

Seeking help when already sober in A.A. is not uncommon, as some symptoms are hidden by alcohol and even by step work or supplements for people in recovery or a temporary scrip for an SSRI. Given time, however, symptoms become manifest and outside help is sought for conditions that come to the fore because we have started to get honest with ourselves. Some see a doctor, others go the emergency room or a hospital. Then the real work begins of finding the right drugs, i.e. medication management, as well as learning about your illness and how to manage side effects, starting therapy or changing it to deal with the new diagnosis and dealing with how this effects sobriety, especially if drugs like Benzos are sometimes needed. It may even be good to find a sponsor who is also a Dualaholic to guide you down that road and any Dual Diagnosis meetings that are available. Sharing about it in a way that is not an outside issue can also be essential in early behavioral recovery and sometimes later.

This type of help was never given to Bill W. when he manifested bipolar symptoms, from promiscuity (the sex thing as other A.A.s would call it) to deep depression. The classic line is that Bill wrote the Twelve and Twelve to get over his depression and gave it to us. In reading one of his biographies, his depression went away when he created the A.A. service structure and gave up running the show as the surviving founder. I felt the same way when I became an elder statesman in AA.

As it stands, it really is already a book on dealing with dual diagnosis, although it has not been marketed as such in A.A. as-a-whole. It is a valid text for any Dualaholic, with some supplementation.

A.A. literature is already full of clues that people can look at to determine if they are alcoholic. The famous pamphlet with ten questions has opened a lot of eyes when people were ready to be honest. With time, most former drunks can answer yes to each question, although at first a few items are in the no category.

Quite a few people now enter A.A. on the blue light special program, meaning they were driving drunk and were pulled over by the police. Whether letting these people come in is a good idea is a matter to be brought up in the discussion of A.A. traditions in a later chapter. Some of these people were just unlucky and not alcoholic. Others, if they are on their second conviction, most likely are (especially if you include deferred sentences), although they might not yet identify in. A few of these people also have mental illness, although driving drunk is not really a symptom of any of the major diagnoses we bring to the behavioral health unit. Still, on the alcoholism side, stories told by both normal alkies and duals can help people who have not hit bottom identify in before their symptoms become obvious.

Early alcoholism is great. You can drink more than anyone else and hangovers are rare. If you avoid driving, you likely will not die (but if you do drive, and have a long way to go, unless you can take a drink with you, the effects will wipe you out before you get home). Many alcoholics learn to drive drunk a bit above speed and never get caught.

Blacking out, can be a problem for some, even in early sobriety. To be clear, blacking out is not falling asleep. It is going full speed ahead with no memory of events. When that happens while you are driving, it could be tragic, or nothing could happen. It depends on how your autopilot works. Very few quit at this stage and, while it would be good for the, it does not seem necessary at the time.

Mid-stage alcoholism can involve drunk driving, unless you rationally give up your vehicle and take cabs. It could interfere with your marriage and children, unless you avoid getting married because it would get in the way of your drinking.

Having a job which can accommodate hangovers or are involved in selling alcohol (including granting you a shift drink) is also typical of a committed alcoholic. A job in politics meets those criteria as well.

Some alcoholics try to cope and may stop on their own or have bad luck and hit an external bottom. Others deliberately lead an alcoholic lifestyle, so they are aware of a problem that they don't want to fix.

Some of these people are Dualaholics for whom drinking is not curative, but it does help control moods or voices. Prescription and street drugs, such as Cannabis, can also fulfill this function.

Late stage alcoholism starts when you can no longer get high. For some, this is when we come in from the cold. Others keep drinking past the point of high tolerance into unpredictability. If they have not yet happened earlier, blackouts may begin, and one is never sure whether taking that drink will cause a blackout, be a night of pointless drinking without catching a buzz or will make you pass out right away. One has to be mentally ill to drink like that but may or may not have a behavioral health diagnosis.

Anyone at that stage won't live long enough to find out, because at that point organs start failing, wet brain starts and bleeding in the stomach and esophagus may result in instant death. Strokes and heart attack are also possible, as they are earlier as well.

These are the lowest bottom drunks, who if they survive can help a lot of newcomers, although at this stage mortality is huge. Any lifeline could be helpful, but many will never take it because it depends on depending on someone other than yourself, even when you can't depend on yourself either. Medical help is definitely essential for these people, but many have been to treatment already and can't see giving it another try. The only possible help is finding some kind of higher power, usually through gratitude, which is a hard sell when your organs are failing.

The alternative to recovery before us is so bleak that, even if we do not believe in God, we still begin to ask Him in the morning to be kept sober that day and to say a thank your prayer each night. Whether we are sincere or fake it until we make it matters not, just do it.

Step Two

*Came to believe that a power greater than ourselves
could restore us to sanity.*

Chapter Four of the *Big Book*, We Agnostics, talks about how one can-find God by opening your mind to the possibility that nature did not create itself, although modern science now seems to think that this is possible. Others are sure that the beauty of nature, from a walk by a lake to a sunlit beach, particularly at dawn, must be evidence of God. Stephen Hawking is grateful that God does not have to exist, but we wonder who he is grateful to for that fact. In the end, it is a personal choice. Does existence cause itself or is it random? In St. Thomas' teaching on the Trinity, are Perfection and Beauty, Truth and Wisdom and Love merely ideas and values or are they living persons in a living God? Again, it is up to you.

Part of any initial answer comes by cultivating gratitude. One need only look a little way back in our drinking, using and mental health careers to see that on many occasions death should have been a certainty other than for the intervention of some active and merciful force. Further, making such a Gratitude List is itself a way to heal anguish and desperation when nothing else is working, when drug interactions have us pacing the floor and where death seems preferable than the present. Yet miraculously, we feel better. Science has shown that for some, there is an attraction to God wired into the brain that does not occur for others, which is either proof of God or proof that spirituality can work for some. Either way, it is good to try what works for now. You can fake it until you make it. There are plenty of A.A.s and probably Duals as well who don't have any of what they call imaginary friends, but they still get better by working the program.

In *Twelve Steps and Twelve Traditions*, Step Two, Bill W. lists all kinds of possible ways drunks relate to God, always with the implication that the cause of our alcoholism came when that relationship was damaged in some way, such as atheism, remorse or anger at God, intellectualism or piety without spirituality.

In this day and age, when the number of Nones and Spiritual but Not Religious (which some copy from A.A. lingo) has grown, largely because people are more honest about not going to Church rather than going for show and social pressure, there has been no epidemic of alcoholism in their ranks. Mental illness either. There are, of course, alcoholic Nones who stopped going as soon as they could, but their genetics or a variety of other causes most likely caused their alcoholism. Others stopped going to Church because they were simply hungover or still drunk to get there. Some with mental illness still find it hard to greet the day on Sunday with a trip to the parish, whether they go to a meeting instead or not. Some go to Yoga. Sunday morning seems a popular time and Yoga can be a good Eleventh Step exercise.

Step Two comes before Step Eleven. It can be taken by believers and non-believers. Indeed, religion is easy to rationalize, to take comfort in and to put on a shelf every Sunday in time for sports or cooking shows (I like the latter). Having a religion does not give one a head-start on this step. It is not enough to have a Higher Power. One must have a Higher Power that will lead you to a spiritual life. Some bit of reeducation is needed. While you must certainly have an idea of God, it needs to be big enough so that you must seek the Truth, rather than thinking you already learned it in Sunday School, CCD, Temple or the Mosque.

Still, Step Two comes after Step One. Being spiritual will not make you a non-alcoholic. For Step Two to make sense, Step One must be complete. You must know that your life is a wreck and Duals need to eventually be aware that stopping drinking is not enough, one must also seek help. Your doctor or therapist is not your higher power either, if it is you are probably drug seeking. God works through these people, but you must be an active consumer, managing and reporting any side effects and doing research, either on your own or through community resources, including fellow Dualaholics. We are not doctors, but we do have experience to share. You must always try to understand what they are giving you. If you ask, doctors will explain, as will pharmacists.

When meds are settling in, as well as during early recovery, attending meetings is crucial to staying grounded as a human being. When it sucks to be you, it is good to have someplace to share that. Step Two is called the "go-to-meetings" step. Doing 90 meetings in 90 days is often recommended. So is doing twice that if you are feeling the urge to drink or are feeling uneasy.

Going to a lot meetings is, along with reading A.A. literature, the best way to immerse yourself in the program. You learn to understand and speak "A.A.". It also gives you someplace to dump the garbage in your mind and soul. You hear about how God is working in the lives of members and that, whatever you thought God was saying to you before, listening to it in the light of what you hear in A.A. might be the wiser course. This is especially true if you thought God said it was OK to drink or to ignore using your psych meds. When it becomes obvious that God was never saying that, sanity begins to return.

For Dualaholics, insanity has more than one meeting. In A.A., the most obvious meaning is drinking when we know what it does to us, thinking that the next time will be different from the last, or if you somehow had a less than ruinous time recently, that such good luck will continue. It never does. That is the nature of alcoholism and the alcoholic obsession.

We have the complication of being truly insane in the sense of a behavioral health diagnosis. When we don't take our meds we are the victims of voices or delusions that we think may come from a higher power when in truth the come from a diseased mind. Some thought us possessed by devils and demons, but that was not the case either. We were just sick.

We are not being persecuted by the President nor tasked by God to end him or her, that is simply a frequent delusion from time immemorial. Most regicides were apolitical, they were just disturbed.

For some of us, mental illness was a useful tool. We were Avant Garde or creative. Many high performing hypomanics are possessed of a genius I.Q. (if there is such a thing), as well as the ability to work intensely, forgoing sleep as an expendable option. Indeed, looking back that lack of a need for sleep was an obvious clue that parents, professors and ourselves should have picked up on, but we kept our own company on such matters.

This does not mean that our lives have been all bad. That manic poetry may be garbage, or it may be very good to some eyes and ears. After years of study, that government reorganization plan may make as much sense as anyone else's. That new way of seeing the economy might be valid. Seeing things that others don't may be insight. Sometimes seeing the obvious is a form of wisdom. The problem was when pain went with it, either psychic or social. Medication, therapy and fellowship can get us past the bad parts and help us to make our contributions useful.

Being diagnosed and finding a community of similar sufferers helps us put both our delusions and successes in perspective. Like non-dual A.A.s, the group is where we hear what God's will really is for us, and that is to be well. We don't necessarily have to be normal, but we can learn to cope with society and behave so that it can cope with us, which is a relief for our families, as we will discuss in Step Nine. This is doubly true for those of us who are Dualaholics. As meeting attendance progresses and we begin to be exposed to a life of faith rather than a life of delusion, we become ready to see the light.

At this point, many newbies think that they may now have a handle on God's will for us. Such thoughts should be run by a sponsor, who should have been procured as early in recovery as possible. Indeed, the first step is not complete until it has been shared, by word or writing, with a sponsor. Sponsors will also assign reading in the *Big Book*, the original 12&12 and maybe this volume. Such reading is very clear. Knowledge of God's will is not available after doing the Second Step. There is much more work to do before arriving at a faith that works, to borrow a phrase from Bill W. To clue you in, Bill was using this phrase in reference to the Eighth and Ninth Steps.

This is also where we begin to pray. We ask every morning to be sober that day and say thanks for that sobriety at night. Whether we do it on our knees, in Lotus, while still in bed, or in walking meditation from our house to the car or bus really does not matter, although some are strident about both praying on your knees and making that bed, the latter being a way to gain some control over our lives. I recommend do the dishes more urgently. The point is to pray, whether you believe in it or not. Fake it until you can. Even if you don't believe in God, making the request changes your life. When you get up or soon after at breakfast, is also a good time to take your meds. What your routine is becomes less important than having one. That you are in a community that keeps the same kind of thing will probably save your life.

Step Three

*Made a decision to turn our will and our lives over
to the care of God, as we understood Him.*

After doing a 90-in-90, most newcomers to A.A. cannot help but wonder about whether their idea of God still worked for them. For most of us, abandoning the thought of a God of vengeance was a natural thing to do. To take this step, it is often enough just to have whatever version we have, even if it is still an A.A. or Dualaholic Group, and go on, as long as that higher power is not us. Being our own higher power is not the road to spirituality. It is the road to delusion. God may live within us but is not us. Once we can appreciate the difference, we can get ready to move on with the program.

We have spent years, if not decades, being our own God. We either escaped an oppressive God of our childhoods or were able to manipulate our understand of God to justify whatever we wanted to do. In recovery, we need to get off that road, whether we were alcoholic, mentally ill or both. Spirituality requires that we learn to seek God's will, not be certain of it based on whatever religiosity we used to possess.

The way to get to an advanced spirituality is to find go through the rest of the Twelve Steps. The Third Step helps us to understand that the way we have been living our lives in disease can no longer be maintained. We cannot use our mental illness to demand more from others than we have a right to expect, whether that mental illness is alcohol and drug abuse or a behavioral health condition. We love to have things our way and being sick takes away our fear of demanding them. Living a spiritual life means getting right-sized.

We cannot control others or stay dependent upon them. Recovery demands that, as much as we can, we must stand on our own two feet. If they are able to help support us, or we are able to gain some type of spiritual support, it is not wrong to accept it, but we cannot use our financial dependence to terrorize our families emotionally, either by domination or dependence.

At this point, we only make the decision to break away. The later steps will help us to heal those relationships and to help others find the resources they need to deal with any codependence that has likely infected their personalities. Sorry, but there is no fellowship for those with relatives who don't take that step for themselves.

As you can see, finding a higher power and a spiritual program is as important for our behavioral health side as it is our alcoholism. Another option is joining Emotions Anonymous and using their literature. Non-alcoholics reading this book should probably keep it for an alcoholic relative and find an EA meeting, as these principles work the best in community. Alcohol is so damaging to our souls, however, that if it is a factor, this is the place to be.

Let's start by unpacking the prayer found in the *Big Book*. "*God, I offer myself to thee, to build with me and do with me as thou wilt.*" My life is a wreck, I can no longer run my life by my rules, I am willing to try yours.

"*Relieve me of the bondage of self, that I may better do they will.*" Selfishness and self-centeredness have got me in their grip. Show me how to live for you because living just for myself has not worked.

"*Take away may difficulties, that victory over them will bear witness to those I would help of Thy Power, thy love and Thy way of life.*" If you help me put my wreck of a life back together, I will help others so that they too can see how this program and works and can work it themselves.

This is the foundation for working the rest of the steps of the program. In the end, the only salvation we have is to help others, but to do so, we have to see how selfishly we are living, because at this stage, we have no idea how bad things really are. This is as true with our mental health as our alcoholism. Indeed, many of our problems are deeper than our drinking and people have been using the A.A. program for them for a long time.

In doing Steps Four and Five, Step Three should be incorporated into the work. When writing an inventory, the Third Step Prayer in the *Big Book* helps to both forestall cravings that may come up with emotions and memories but will also help us to continue writing. Note that the Prayer does not contain the word Alcohol, so there is no reason to ignore its usefulness on the behavioral health side as well, just as the effect of dependence is the same for both conditions.

In Step Five, we say the prayer with our sponsors, as we may have when first taking Step Three, to bring God into that event. More about that later.

The Third Step does not ask God to give us recovery on a silver platter. It is just the opposite. God is asked to give us strength and guidance while WE do a fearless moral inventory, then WE share this inventory with God and our sponsor. These steps make us ready to have God remove these defects of character. It is only in Step Seven, as we will explain, that we begin to notice miracles in our lives beyond simply keeping us sober.

Step Three is our becoming willing to do these things, not have them done for us. We take it when we are ready to work. When not working to improve our characters and depend on God is more painful than making the effort to take these steps.

The reason for this book is that a spiritual awakening through dependence on a higher power, including using that power as a way to overcome defects of character is not something most therapists are comfortable dealing with, unless they are also twelfth steppers. A therapeutic model which ignores these factors will not prove as effective when the chips are down as membership in a twelfth step fellowship and acceptance of both our defects of character and our powerlessness of dealing with them on our own.

Therapists who try to sugarcoat what must be done are not helping Dualaholics get better. A spiritual program, even for confirmed agnostics, is better than years of therapy, which has its place, but cannot do what a fellowship with a spiritual program can. Dualaholics are lucky losers because we have access to such a program. Seeing the program from the standpoint of mental health recovery will show how much more useful it can be.

The Third Step is not an invitation to the delusion that we know God's will, which therapists are leery of Dualaholics doing, but is rather a way to subject ourselves to Him, and probably for the first time in our lives, live in humility in relation to God or reality or whatever power you need to relate yourself to that is greater than yourself.

It is important here to emphasize that we do not know God's will just because we have said the Third Step Prayer, although the prayer does give us a strong hint that it involves helping others and getting out of our own heads. We have merely asked, but as yet have no ability to hear the answer. If you think you know God's will at Step Three, the answer is most surely No, you don't.

Nothing is more vexing than a newcomer who thinks that saying the prayer gives them divine knowledge. That supposed knowledge is the past calling, usually to come home and see the wife and kids or take the old job back. Until Steps Four through Nine are attempted, no newcomer to either alcoholic or behavioral recovery should face the past unaided. Stay in recovery living as long as possible until these steps are complete. When you develop a healthy fear in these areas, you may be ready, but first, fearlessly write the Fourth Step.

Step Four

Made a searching and fearless moral inventory of ourselves.

There are many ways to do a Fourth Step inventory. The *Big Book* contains a chart that focuses on our relationships. The *Twelve & Twelve* has questions and also directs us to chart our relationships. Back to Basics has an easy to fill in matrix (it almost does itself). Hazelden has products for both Alcoholics (The Red Book) and Dualaholics. The problem with the last two is that they were done for us, not by us. The whole premise of the Fellowship is that we are doing our own program, mostly because we don't listen to outsiders who want to tell us how to get sober without doing it themselves. There are other inventories that come with later steps, but for now, let us focus on this one. Always remember that whatever tool you use, you will be writing about your favorite subject, yourself, although this time you must be honest.

The classic inventory is still the one from the *Big Book*. You begin with a pad of paper (or an Access, Work, or Excel table) and first list everyone you resent, as well as institutions and idea. This is actually better for Dualaholics, because we both have a lot of resentments and many of them are with or at people that we don't know, from the President to the Pope to the judges on American Idol. In some cases, we know that they are distant, in others we have the delusion of familiarity with those we resent. Those people should be listed.

We then go down the list and say why we resent them (so leave a few lines between each name or use that software). This may be where we start to really become aware of the level of fantasy in our lives. It is also where we use the Third Step readings, from the chapter above to the *Big Book*, to get some perspective. The reality is that we are not that different in our delusions and our desire to force the world into the way we want it than any "normal" alcoholic. At this stage, we gentle with ourselves. The temptation to escape back to the bottle, extra meds or street drugs or other acting out is strong. Pray for strength as required and stay in touch with your sponsor as you go through this.

Next, we list what area the relationship is in. The standard three are sex, society and security, which is divided into financial and personal relationships. You can use more than one and I would add delusion to cover those people where the relationship was all in our minds. That can be the high school crush you never spoke to or the President. If you are using a database or table, this is a good place for check boxes.

Finally, we list our part. In almost every Club that holds meetings there is some kind of listing of character defects. There are probably too many options, but if you desire many, leave field open. If not, a two-column table in this cell could name the seven deadly sins of pride, greed, lust, anger, gluttony, envy and sloth, with the addition of fear. If you use these boxes (or put them in the header), please feel free to check more than one.

The *Big Book* has a few prayers for doing the inventory, especially when you write down people you really did behave badly as well. Pray for them as a sick person. Anything to let go.

Next comes the matter of fear. This is a good thing for all Behavioral Health patients to face. You could even rate the fears one to ten with ten being realistic and one being fantasy or delusion. This can be a turning point in living your life.

Both therapists and Bill W. in the Twelve & Twelve recommended pointing out character assets. This does not counter-act the defects list, which has a purpose and is not meant to be a downer. This is a good place to list them, right after the fears and maybe even with the same one-to-ten ranking so that we are honest with ourselves about any delusions.

Next comes the sex inventory on page 69. I had an older sponsee who tells the story of some (it may have been him) who read the instructions from page 96 on recruiting newcomers during a step study on this inventory. I invite you to give it a look and see why it is funny.

The *Big Book* does not offer much advice on a sex inventory other than listing victims, which is important, although more a matter for Step Eight, and developing sexual ideal. This did not do Bill W. much good. As a Bipolar sufferer, he had a lot of trouble with casual and non-casual affairs. Medication would have helped and probably therapy. What ultimately worked for him were the questions he developed in the *Twelve*

& Twelve as they related to sex. Use them (and any of the others that pertain to you, but especially the sex questions).

Some questions are in order for those Dualaholics who have special sexual issues, such as transition. We are not trying to be nosy or talk you out of doing something you have always known is right for you, however doing this inventory first, as well as the following steps, is urgent so that you don't make an unchangeable decision based on a feeling of apartness or uncomfortablity without exploring the fact that all Dualaholics have such feelings in some measure. Make sure you are squared away spiritually before they start using scalpels.

Asking yourself the question if your uncomfortably with your gender or other sexual identity issues is because of a mistake in nature or is part of your Dualaholic nature is critical, as many are unsatisfied after the process and end up ending themselves. We will love you in either gender, but we don't want to bury you just yet.

Getting spiritual does not mean you can't still be delightfully outrageous, by the way. It is good, however, to be able to control the volume. None of us got sober to stop having fun. We simply want to have the fun rather than the fun having us.

Finishing your inventory can be scary, because the next stop is sharing it with a sponsor, therapist, spiritual leader or all of the above. This is a time to go to more meetings and pray more, because the next steps are the most transformative of your life and probably more effective in it than any therapy you have ever had.

Step Five

*Admitted to God, to Ourselves and to Another
Human Being the Exact Nature of Our Wrongs.*

This is one point in recovery where you will want to drink, use or up your meds to deal with the pressure of having done a fearless and thorough moral inventory and realize that you are about to share it. If you pray, this is when to do it. Do not despair, everyone feels a bit of fear at this point, but working through that fear and sharing what you have written is one of the best moments of your life.

If you believe in religious confession, you should certainly share it with a confessor if he knows about alcoholism and mental illness, but make appointment. This takes more time than is available when others are waiting in line. Likewise, this may take more time than the standard therapy appointment. Also, you don't want this in your medical file, but you can certainly share the highlights and how the step went, although if you really trust your therapist you can talk about it before your sponsor. Sharing with your sponsor, however, is where you really feel like you are a member of A.A. or any Dualaholic fellowship, if only because your sponsor has things to share from their experience that will put you at ease, especially if they also have mental illness.

As stated previously, you begin with the Third Step Prayer, which invokes the presence of God (who is there anyway, but the prayer helps you know it). Often, you then get the most embarrassing thing out of the way, which you will find is not that uncommon, even for Dualaholics. Your sponsor will talk you through the rest. There will be some things he or she will tell you not to worry about and others that will be emphasized, usually regarding those closest to you. Before long it is easy to continue, because you are talking about your favorite subject, you, but by now in a loving way.

If you are depressed, this is quite a breakthrough. It is not unlike Cognitive Behavioral Therapy, except it happens all at once and sets the groundwork for methods that CBT will never touch. If you are grandiose, this will put your delusions in perspective, but gently. We all have both sides and, in truth, being constantly down on yourself is still an egocentric exercise. The care of a fellow sufferer will show that these problems can and have been solved and will be for you.

When you reach the end, the topic of what comes next will arise. If you have a good sponsor, there will be more and better directions than letting the steps work you. For Dualaholics, there may be things to share with your therapist or doctor. If there are criminal matters to-discuss, this is not the time to take action. That is the Eighth and Ninth Steps. In most, if not all, jurisdictions what you share in your inventory is privileged. The main instructions will be to go ahead and do Steps Six and Seven, as described in the *Big Book*. These instructions are as applicable to Dualaholics as any other A.A.

Dualaholics are outsiders by nature. Once you have done his step, you will find that this feeling has gone away. While our traditions state that you are a member because you say you are, you really feel like it once you have done this step. You are no longer an isolated freak or sinner, but instead a full member of the human race. There are no perfect people or perfectly flawed people. We are all in the middle someplace and you have officially joined the group by experiencing this step. (Sorry, but reading about it in this book is not enough).

Knowing that even though you are a Dualaholic, which means you are more than a little insane, that accepting it gives you freedom, a freedom that we give to each other more profound than anything we can get in therapy.

Step Six

*Were entirely ready to have God remove all these
defects of character.*

Note the wording of this step. It does not say our sponsor, our therapist or doctor or ourselves. It says God. There are people who, when they say the serenity prayer, say "others" after the first part and "me" after the second. The second is a fool's errand. We are powerless over everything, including the characters we are born with. What we can choose to change is how we respond to situations, but whether it is conditioning, astrology or genetics that gives us our characters, they are hard-wired without divine intervention. This is not as mysterious as it sounds. If we try to fix ourselves, we are thinking about ourselves again. If we think about others or about what God wants for them, then we have more of a reason to act rightly. Egocentrism just does not do the job.

In the *Big Book*, we are instructed in Step Six to go home and meditate on the first five steps to examine if we have done them thoroughly and are then ready to move along with the program. Since that looks like a yes and no question, it does not take the hour prescribed, although you could read either this book or the *Twelve & Twelve* chapters to eat the time. You could also say the Seventh Step Prayer and make your amends list (it really only takes an hour to do so).

You could read this chapter (you are certainly doing that now, or is this statement false? or is it true? Sorry, but you just did your Step Five and needed a joke and remember that the author of this book is a Dualaholic and therefore insane). You could read the Step Six Chapter in the *Twelve & Twelve*. Both chapters agree that Step Six takes more than an hour (and you should still do that hour of meditation and say the Prayer). These are lifetime adventures.

In the *Twelve & Twelve*, Bill W. goes on a journey through the seven deadly sins, from the ones that constitute major violations of human conduct, like rape and murder, which are avoided out of self-preservation, to more minor character flaws, like taking our comfort, which is an outdated way of saying treating ourselves or having it our way.

What he was attacking was the impurity of our motives and the need to point at sub level toward the most pure of motives, which is seeking the perfection of God. Of course, if we were to find it on those terms would really mess up our humility. His point was that we needed to constantly strive for that kind of perfection, which was one of the goals of the Oxford Movement that he and Dr. Bob came out of (not to be confused with Oxford Houses). Sandy B. related in a talk at Sessions that when the Twelve was published Bill went to Bob's grave in Akron and told him he had put perfection back in the program.

This is where alcoholics, dualaholics and therapists start complaining that such a program is unattainable and it plays right into the hands of the depressive side of our disease. They are half right, but it gets worse.

The perfection of God is not really about having perfect conduct or perfectly avoiding sin. That would be self-centered in the extreme, also obsessive compulsive. No, the real perfection, which there is not excuse but to strive for is the perfection of God where God is perfect, which is prefect Love. Loving others perfectly is a lot harder than simply not offending them, or God (who as God, really cannot be hurt by human conduct anyway).

It is a side effect that showing perfect love for other people results in not sinning against them, although if you have a sponsee who is killing themselves, directly or with substances, not offending them would get in the way of saving their lives.

If we lived alone on desert islands, we would have no character defects. No one would be affected by our actions. Living in society means we must consider our obligations to others, especially to love them.

The point of Step Six is to become ready to ask God to do something that we cannot do by any kind of therapy or practice, to give us the willingness to love everyone perfectly, as He loves them.

Step Seven

Humbly asked Him to remove our shortcomings.

Note well that this step does not say we fixed ourselves. Indeed, we are not even good at telling what is broken, even after doing inventory and resolving to love others perfectly. Unpacking the prayer, which is all the *Big Book* says about Step Seven, helps us see this.

"My Creator, I am now will that you shall have all of me, good and bad." We give ourselves to the care of God, as we did when we started to clean house.

"I ask you now to remove all these defects of character that stand in the way of my usefulness to you and my fellows." We simply don't know which character traits will be helpful and which get in the way of helping others. This is as true for behavioral issues as it is for alcoholism. False humility can be as toxic as false pride. We must trust God to help us.

"Grant me strength as I go out from here to do your bidding." We do not ask for God's help to make us meek or weak, but to make us useful to others, both other alcoholics, other behavioral health patients and especially those who are both, as well as the other people in our lives who we have impacted or will impact.

There is nothing that mental health practitioners should find objectionable, it is just that sharing faith is not something that they can do unless they are fellow sufferers. Some in ministry might help if they have the mental health knowledge and are as interested in saving our asses as our souls.

So, the question is, does this work? Recovered alcoholics, addicts and dualaholics will universally say yes. While sometimes the first part of the removal of a defect is noticing how much it hurts, taking it to God has awesome consequences. Addictions to gluttony, pornography, gossip, aggressive driving and spitefulness seem to melt away for the asking, provided we ask humbly, and even when we have not. Some of us find ourselves in the center lane of traffic going with the flow and marvel at how fast we aren't going in attempts to pass everyone on the freeway.

Defects we used to use as comfort suddenly lose their appeal. We simply tire of them. If we are in A.A. Service, we realize that maybe that resolution we were pushing at the Area Assembly can wait a bit. Miracles simply happen and we open our hearts to other people when our lives have previously been isolation.

Do we do all of this alone? No. We can use sponsors, especially when lingering defects cause us pain, as well as therapists and counselors who have valuable tools, like affirmations and cognitive behavioral therapy that help us deal with toxic thoughts. There is no harm in trying anything that works.

We certainly do not stop taking our medications because God is helping us with our characters. This step does not say that we humbly asked Him to make our minds whole. At best, this may help us work toward more accurate diagnosis or have the courage to ask our doctors to stop medications where the side effects are too great for us to bear.

As the *Twelve & Twelve* states, our relationship to humility changes. What was like fear and humiliation becomes more like trust. Like the entire book, which was written around Bill W.'s mental illness, this chapter is particularly full of profound truths. He states that humility will be something we desire. This idea takes some getting used to, as well as his statement that the difference between a request and a demand should be simple for everyone to see. He did not say the obvious, which is everyone but alcoholics seem to know. I once noted this and a sponsee, who had more than twice the time I did, agreed and started using it in his share too. The punch line is that it is God who helps us see the difference with time.

Desiring humility seems hard until you define what humility is. Some say it not thinking less about yourself, but thinking about yourself less. Of course, as Buckaroo Banzai pointed out, "no matter where you go, there you are." Also heard at meetings was that humility is accepting yourself exactly as you are and exactly as you aren't. That corresponds to a definition of Love that exists in the motivational community, to accept yourself or the other person in the same way. Again, this ties the humility we seek to God's perfect love and our desire to both experience and share that love. We cannot do this on our own, we must ask with whatever humility we have. It certainly is not perfect at this stage.

There is nothing in this standard of either humility or love that makes it incompatible with recovery from mental illness. Indeed, self-acceptance is a major goal. It is vitally necessary to achieve it before we can heal and repair our relationships with others. Of course, until we examine those relationships by doing an inventory in Step Four, we cannot begin either task.

This step is a life-long endeavor. We never master it nor does God seek to make us perfect in our conduct. This could only happen in his Perfect Direct Presence, which is found nowhere on earth. We must make due with freedom and with asking for His help (or Her's if we are talking about the Spirit, which in Christianity is Love). Without freedom, we could never seek God's help, but be doomed to make the same mistakes over and over again, as we did when we were drinking, using or controlled by our symptoms.

Our life long journey toward humility and love does start with that first time we say the Seventh Step Prayer, the night we come home after sharing our inventory with a sponsor and deciding that we were willing. We are now ready to keep moving along with-the program, for the Prayer strengthens us for the journey.

Some people ask if we put our own names on the amends list in Step Eight. We think not. Step Seven is where we make our amends to ourselves by asking God to heal us, so that we may love ourselves exactly as we are and exactly as we aren't. What better amend is there than that? What better affirmation than requesting the help of a power greater than ourselves?

Step Eight

Made a list of all persons we had harmed and became willing to make amends to them all.

In this step we take our self-centered moral inventories and turn them to a list of amends we have to make to help make ourselves whole. The secret to this step and the next is that God fixes our defects of character by putting us in contact with other people with whom those defects were active. How this happens comes in Step Nine, but the need to get to that step is vital if we are to become fully functioning human beings.

Early on the Inventory was used as the amends list. No separate writing was required, just the willingness to make amends and the discussion with a sponsor on how to do so. Back when A.A. was young, lists did not get as long as they do now, especially for today's self-centered alcoholics and dualaholics. Whether the people on our lists where the entire relationship is delusional should be included or not is also a matter we take up with our sponsors. We can certainly pray for them but leaving them off is as valid a strategy for moving away from fantasy.

Today, we usually write a separate list, with categories like direct amends, living amends, financial amends and letters, both mailed and unmailed. Some even divide the list to those where we are-willing to take action and those where it will take some time.

As the *Twelve & Twelve* says, forgiveness is a big part of adding someone to an amends list. While many people did us some kind of harm, especially the emotional kind, it is likely because our alcoholic, addict and mentally twisted conduct drove them away or caused a bad reaction. When we were sick, whether needy or acting out, we were not pleasant to be around and must be grateful to any that did not run away from fear, and probably to those who did before we could hurt them even worse. No one needed our permission to protect themselves emotionally or even physically.

There is, of course, the truism that we attract people like ourselves, even in recovery. How many children of alcoholics have been lured into relationships where their past becomes alive, even if they and we have been in recovery? Still, we cannot demand their allegiance just because we are finally feeling better. Remember that in Step Seven we accepted ourselves exactly the way we were and exactly the way we were not, knowing that God has already done the same. How can we deny that acceptance to everyone we have encountered in our lives, near and far. Indeed, if we do this right, it no longer becomes about us at all. As we try living by such a credo, we get a glimpse of the perfect love we must have for others that is the essential part of Step Six.

The amends we propose should bear some relation to the harm we did and the character change we need to make. Don't get too attached to the amend proposed, however, because before you do anything, you must have your sponsor look at what you have written. Failure to do that could be disastrous. Under his direction, you may also want to consult your therapist and, if violations of law have occurred, your attorney.

Everything the *Big Book* and *Twelve & Twelve* say about caution in burdening spouses with the knowledge of affairs they did not know about or reporting yourself for crimes committed, petty and major, applies to Dualaholics. We generally will not tell you to turn yourself in to the boss or the police without a great deal of consultation, especially for matters most serious. It may be that your own sense of justice will drive you in that direction, but do not act as recklessly in planning amends as you did in causing harm. That is not recovery, it is the same conduct repeated.

Most of us, by the grace of God, don't have issues that major. Still, we bring our list to our sponsors. He will likely change many amends, especially the self-centered and dramatic ones and will likely tell you to ignore people from your distant past, even if putting them on the list was helpful. For the living amends, there will be suggestions on how to be more fully functional, suggestions your therapist will likely agree with. Most of us need the input from both, but the sponsor has the experience in living a spiritual life despite both having both diseases, and in this case, experience matters. This is where we pass from early to long term recovery. We make our amends, track them and continue inventory, pray and begin to help other alcoholics. We are ready for the second part of our adventure, where we really learn to depend on God.

Step Nine

Made direct amends to such people wherever possible, except when to do so would injure the or others.

Aside from getting clean and sober and going on medication, this is the most visible outward manifestation of our recoveries. In making our amends, we begin to change our lives to become or return to some kind of normality. We go to school or get some kind of employment, either again or for the first time. We may apply for disability assistance or some kind of assisted housing or else find housing on our own. We may participate in a treatment or psychiatric rehabilitation program. We work on ourselves. We might even, when we are ready, look for a healthy relationship, one which does not involve codependence. We begin to stand on our own two feet, which is a living amends to those who have helped us.

In order to repair our reputations, we may have made direct amends to past employers, schools and neighbors. We especially take care to appreciate people in our families who have and will continue to be our support network, whose fondest desire is for us to be well. We involvement in our crisis management plans and keep these up to date.

We continue to go to meetings and our active in the fellowship, welcoming newcomers, doing service and participating in meetings. We begin to wear our dualaholic recovery like a loose garment. After a few years, we may even participate in service above the group level at intergroup, the district and area. We give what was so freely given to us.

Of course, none of this is easy. Sometimes getting out of the house is still hard, but if we can, we do it anyway. We also follow our sponsors' directions in making amends. We don't get into arguments or make amends that may harm those we would seek to grow closer too, especially if doing so would really hurt them. Some things need to remain secret, but we make these decisions with the help of both sponsors and therapists, and possibly attorneys.

We never brag about our illnesses to Normies who would be dismayed by our stories. When a parent insists you were not that bad, do not argue and reveal how bad you were. This is not the time to make an argument or brag. Your mother does not need to know that you sold drugs or your own body. At the same time, be ready to answer any questions they have, but reserve the right to not answer right away or ever if it is too painful.

You may mention resources in the community or in Al Anon Family Groups or Alcoholics Anonymous that may be helpful to them, but we don't force recovery on anyone.

If your marriage is ending, you behave like an adult. You don't hold onto what was lost, nor stalk an ex-spouse or romantic partner. If children are involved and you were a source of trauma, it may take years to make things right. Do not rush it. You have a lifetime to work things out although you don't have the right to expect that they will. Leave some things in God's hands. Seek professional help when appropriate or step away as needed.

This is the time when the Promises begin to come true and you realize you have gained God consciousness. Usually this is because, regardless of your plans, the amends you make show up on the Divine schedule rather than your own. When this happens, make the amend if you are able. You will find them easier than you feared. If you are reading this, remember that this is a process that happens with and to you. Reading about it is not enough to make the promises come true. You must experience all of the steps to have them work. It is a program of action, not education. You cannot just talk it through with your sponsor or therapist or in a step group. You have to do it. It is a lifelong endeavor.

Step Ten

Continued to take personal inventory and when we were wrong, promptly admitted it.

This is the Do-Over step. It saves us because we are not always on the beam. Sometimes we fall off and this step helps us back on. It works whether others are mad at us or we are mad at them, because if we are angry, it includes our unreasonable expectations of others to give us what we want on our terms. When we admit to doing that, we humanize ourselves in the eyes of others, finally behaving as adults, and they often become fast friends.

Some people wait for upset to occur before doing this step, although that may be too late if there are parts of our life that are chronically upset in relationships at home or work or in the community. If we wait for a blowup, it may be too late to make things right. People who were never fired when drinking or in mental health disease sometimes find themselves losing jobs that they could have kept and would have if the job enabled our using or illness.

The *Big Book* contains questions for nightly inventory in the Tenth Step section and for a morning inventory in the Eleventh. Likewise, there are suggested meditations in both sections. The idea of ever facing any kind of inventory without involving a Higher Power should fill anyone with fear, both for the experience and the result, which would be sadly incomplete. It is the kind of old behavior we should avoid at all costs and if done holistically is the key to emotional sobriety.

Dualaholics who got sober with or after their mental health diagnosis will be able to combine their mental health and addiction Fourth and Fifth Step work at the same time. Those who were diagnosed after they got sober can chose to do a full Fourth and Fifth Steps or can do a Tenth Step inventory instead. It is likely that many of the people who would be on such an inventory were on the original inventory and on the living amends list. They may have been relatives who had been insisting that more was wrong than just alcoholism. For these people, letting them say I told you so as they visit you in the hospital is a justified bit of humble pie.

The *Twelve & Twelve* also inter-relates mediation, inventory and prayer as the secret to emotion sobriety. Indeed, such an exercise is said to have pulled Bill W. out his depression, when he had few options in terms of medication. Meditating on the St. Francis Prayer, also known as the Prayer for Peace, was key to this. It is also useful to use this prayer as a written recovery. Many of the items in the prayer are very good for an examination of ones ideas on personal importance and even grandiosity. As such, it is a good exercise for Dualaholics. It is not harsh, but it is a good mirror that can be used therapeutically.

There are all sorts of personality inventories out there for mental health patients and they should be used diagnostically, however for gaining power over our diseases so that we may act rightly, those based on A.A. literature seem most appropriate, at least if they are to be used in A.A. meetings or with an A.A. sponsor. Therapists who are also in recovery have a sense of this already and if they find a good product, by all means, use it. We also suggest that you use these well.

It may seem that I have left nothing else to talk about for the Eleventh Step. That is not the case. There is a wealth of topics and ideas for Dualaholics to use in seeking a more normal life.

Step Eleven

Sought through prayer and meditation to improve our conscience contact with God, as we understood Him, praying only for knowledge of his will for us and the power to carry that out.

We have already spoken about meditation as a tool to be used with inventory as a tool to work for emotional sobriety. Meditation can also be used for both physical and spiritual sobriety, sometimes at the same time. People with mental illness of all types hyperventilate on occasion, either as a separate problem or as part of a panic episode.

Controlled breathing of all types, as well as rescue medications, are parts of the solution. To fall asleep quickly, the classic is four counts in, hold seven, eight out, and repeated as necessary. Of course, this is for sleep and not panic and for some it is too harsh (by some, I include myself). Ten in, ten hold and ten out is what my sponsor recommends and those who practice Yoga know about full yogic breathing which goes from the stomach and diaphragm to the lungs and then back in reverse. Yogis recommend all breathing through the nose, while others inhale through the nose and exhale through the mouth. What you use depends on how you are taught.

Spiritual sobriety can certainly be pursued with outside help, either from the religion of your childhood, an adult conversion or an eastern meditation or yogic practice. Use whatever you find comfortable. If it sings to you and offers you hope, then use it, but be a critical user. While you are of course free to follow your faith, we suggest you avoid those meditations that threaten Hell, as you have already been there and the program is an attempt for you to not go back.

While inventory and mediation are comfortable territory for therapists, prayer really is not. Indeed, spiritual prayer is not really understood by many clergy, save the Jesuits who follow a similar spiritual path (indeed, we follow them rather than their following us). At this stage, you get to choose your path.

You are also free to pray as your like. but we suggest you free yourself from your old ways of prayer. Prayer is not magic which we use to bribe God. God's will happens in God's time, regardless of the thoughts and prayers we send his way. Praying for others most likely does not change their fates, but it may change how we think and act in relation to them, especially if tragedy has occurred and bringing a casserole dish is appropriate. It is an act of solidarity, which puts us all on a more spiritual plain.

Growing up, some of us were told to pray for multiple things, like vocations to the religious life or our national leaders or for some classmate's sick parent or dead grandparent. While there is nothing wrong with these prayers, they become a chore that likely take us off praying. In A.A., as we learn to pray spiritually, it becomes less of a chore and more of an opportunity to actually speak intimately with God.

Instead of telling God what we want for ourselves, we ask him what he wants from us next. We don't do this without knowledge of our talents and hopes, we affirm that we will do what He bids rather than powering through our lives on self-will. If your prayers seem to be getting grandiose, you may want to share them with a sponsor, doctor or therapist, but if your medications are in order and you are following these directions and those in A.A. literature, you will likely be doing OK.

We will soon be ready to really know God's will for us (let His will for others be His secret) and we seek strength to go down the road that we see when spiritually awake. Indeed, we are much more awake than previously. As we do our amends, our ability to see God's will becomes more acute. It is in the next step where we find ourselves as awake as we can be, finally knowing what God's will for us actually is. (The title of the Step gives it away.)

Step Twelve

Having had a Spiritual Awakening as the result of these steps, we tried to carry this message to Alcoholics and to practice these principles in all our affairs.

Remember back when we took the Third Step prayer and wondered how we knew God's will? We're here. We have had some inkling as the promises began to come true after we had begun our Step Nine amends, which seemed to have a life of their own. Now we are sure, because this step tells us. God's will for us is to try to carry this message to Alcoholics and to practice these principles in all of our affairs. The latter means that we treat everyone, family member or stranger, as if they were fellow members of A.A.. Indeed, our lives depend on our do. Backsliding on loving everyone as God loves them can lead us back to the bottle and a quick or a long painful death. Since God does not want our suicide by alcohol, drugs or our own hand, doing His will is essential.

How we got there is reiterated in a very long paragraph in the Step Twelve chapter of the *Twelve & Twelve*. What we must do to stay awake is to give this program away, both at meetings and by finding people to sponsor and passing on what we have been given. Indeed, we may find ourselves telling sponsees things we have heard at meetings that we never thought we would say, especially when they tell us they may be thirsty. We may talk much more firmly than we ever thought we would, but that it is because God is talking through us and we are this person's only hope in that moment. Other times, we find ourselves far more compassionate than we thought capable. Again, God is speaking through us, not because we mediated and decided what to say but because we felt inspired to say it in the moment. That is what being spiritually awake looks like and our health care providers need not have any fear that we have gone round the bend. We have not.

We cannot exercise such spiritual power without making ourselves ready by doing the Steps before. In fact, taking our chargees through the Steps is our job as Sponsor. While anyone can make an A.A. friend by giving their ear and reassurance to a newcomer, that is a far cry from what sponsors do. There is a ton of A.A. literature about it in the pamphlet about sponsorship, the *Big Book* and the *Twelve & Twelve*. Of course, the best source is your own sponsor, especially if he or she is a fellow Dualaholic.

Of course, most people find their sponsors at meetings, as well as their first service commitment, usually coffee maker or secretary. After a while, they may have enough time to be group chair, if that is a separate thing. If it is not, then waiting until you are six months in to be secretary is sound advice, or at least what we did in the past. Many groups who consider such things also prefer that people have six months to lead the meeting (aka qualify).

Of late, it has been fashionable for qualifiers to give a long drunkalog but little comment on how they worked the steps (many have not) and what it is like now (if they have not worked the steps, it's not a pretty picture). That kind of lead is mainly for anniversary meetings, not discussion or step meetings (it used to be that only speaker meetings were open so that members could share their complete names, as we are not anonymous from each other).

In open discussion meetings, the leader will briefly qualify, share a bit about a topic appropriate to a meeting with non-members, such as gratitude and then open it up for sharing after ten minutes, usually fifteen minutes into the meeting. In the old days, the leader would comment between shares. We will talk about what is shared regarding Traditions Five and Six. One thing we don't do is let abusive shares continue, nor is bragging about using or hurting someone allowed, as it disturbs A.A. Unity, see Tradition One.

In step meetings, we read the step chapter or section of the *Big Book* and someone who did the step may make a few remarks then open it up for sharing by people who have done the step. Those who have not can speak up and share if they have a burning desire to do so.

A few updates on practicing these principles in all our affairs. The economy has now become as bad as it was when the *Big Book* was written, so bankruptcy is more widely used, especially by those of us with more than a few mental health hospitalizations that happened before we were put on Medicaid. Combine that with underwater mortgages (although things are looking up) and credit card debt at high rates and there is no shame in either working our way out of debt or throwing in the towel. It is not very spiritual, however, to make a habit of it so we try to get some kind of coverage as we can afford it. We don't stand in our pride in apply for assistance if it means our medical team gets paid, or we even get to have a medical team.

If families offer help, we take it for a bit, but we try to get on our feet as soon as possible, especially if we can qualify for long term disability, which is also the access to discharging student loans, especially if we did not finish or cannot use the degree. We also try to find day programs so that our families are not burdened with our presences. Sloth is an easy defect if we have nothing else to do. That can make a working spouse upset, even if we are having a medication reaction that confines us to bed.

If we have the energy to work and our heads are relatively clear, this is an option to look at. In 2008, many people were given disability as jobs were almost impossible to get. They are no longer impossible, so it may be a good time to make the effort. States have offices that help us do that.

Sometimes the family dynamic is broken by our multiple problems. Unlike when the *Twelve & Twelve* were written, divorce in A.A. and among behavioral health patients has become quite common. We do not begrudge our spouses their freedom if they must leave. It was likely not an easy decision for them or their support structures (at least we hope not). We do not stalk them, threaten them or hold out hope that they will return, although some do anyway. Likewise, unless they are sicker than we are, we let them dictate how to deal with the children. The law gives us certain rights to both custody and assets and spirituality does not require that we give these up, as making normal arrangements allows us to not be a burden on our parents and siblings. Also, we don't head to the Altar or Justice of the Peace with the first person we meet just because we are lonely or to rub our spouses' noses in it. Doing so seems to be a sure way to get drunk.

The *Twelve & Twelve* mentioned people who could not have a family as providing prodigies of service to A.A. as a whole. Bill was talking about our LGBT brothers and sisters, who did and still do join in service. People with families do as well, especially if the families have two incomes. Also, our LGBT folk can now have the same family concerns that we do, though that won't keep them out of service.

This is the Service that was described as a solution to our problems of personal importance, our still wanting to be President or even running a few times (which Americans Elect allowed some of us to do until it realized who was running). In helping A.A. govern itself, we do find that we don't need to necessarily share our opinions as much as we would or have our motion pass by force of will. We also find the strength to speak up if we otherwise wouldn't. Of course, some of us do throw our two cents in often, but if we have something that needs to be said, that may be God using us despite our defects as we say in the Seventh Step Prayer. Of course, if those problems persist, we will also discuss them with our sponsor, our therapist and our doctor, but the side effects of such medication changes should be watched closely.

What Bill was referring to by prodigies of Service are another part of the Twelfth having to do with Service above the group level (note the capital S), which has to do with the Ninth Tradition, where we set up service committees (Districts, Area Assemblies, the General Service Conference which decides A.A. issues), all of which are responsible to the A.A. Group through your Group Services Representative (which we will talk about in the Fourth Tradition). Indeed, much of the Twelfth Step happens regarding the Traditions and the Service Structure that lives within them. It is where we have A.A. Phone Lines, Hospital and Institution Commitments and all the ways we carry the message more systematically than meetings. We still have much more to talk about.

The Traditions

We will discuss the Traditions as they related to Dualaholic in or outside of A.A. in a few paragraphs each. See the *Twelve & Twelve* for a more complete discussion off A.A. Tradition.

Tradition One

Our common welfare should come first: personal recovery depends upon A.A. Unity.

The Dualaholic movement is very small. Indeed, most of us don't attend special meetings and rarely discuss problems associated with mental illness in the meetings they do go to. This book raises the question on whether we become more visible or continue mostly in shadows. Is hiding good for A.A. Unity, should we be a constituent group, like those for sex or sexual orientation or should we become a separate fellowship? More will be revealed.

Tradition Two

For our group purpose there is but one ultimate authority--a loving God as he may express Himself in our group conscience. Our leaders are but trusted servants; they do not govern.

Our group conscience includes us, either as A.A. members or as Dualaholics, whether in standard groups, Dualaholics groups or a separate fellowship. It does not include our doctors, therapists, treatment centers or non-member authors.

Tradition Three

The only requirement for A.A. membership is a desire to stop drinking.

This means that if you are an alcoholic with a mental illness, you are welcome in A.A. If you are dual-addicted, you are welcome in A.A. (as Bill W. once wrote in the A.A. Grapevine). If you are an addict without alcoholism, Bill suggested you not share because it is confusing to newcomers who need an alcoholic message to identify in. This raises the question of whether Dualaholics should share at A.A. meetings. Since Bill W. wrote the *Twelve & Twelve* to work on his mental health issues and is known to have been bipolar, we suspect the answer is yes. In Dualaholics meetings, if an addict is also mentally ill, the answer is maybe, but we think it is probably yes, especially if a separate fellowship is formed. Emotions Anonymous is also an option if they allow sharing on alcoholism.

Tradition Four

Each group should be autonomous except in matters affecting other groups or A.A. as a whole.

This means that we can probably have our own meetings, although whether these should have a Group Services Representative, a Group Number and contribute money to any Central Office, as well as the General Service Board is an evolving question that does affect A.A. as a whole. We would not be considered under "Treatment" because we are part of the Fellowship. Because there are now a few member-created books, it is likely that the Literature Committee will also be involved.

Tradition Five

Each group has but one primary purpose—to carry its message to the alcoholic who still suffers.

Dualaholics are alcoholics who still suffer, as are the dual-addicted, according to Bill W. We definitely need the message, as this volume shows with its frequent instruction to use A.A. literature in completing the steps.

Let us remember that the Tradition Five chapter in the *Twelve & Twelve* does not mention use of narcotics. It illustrated why we have no religious affiliation (save renting basements). There is no Catholic A.A., Evangelical A.A., Jewish A.A. or Muslim A.A., no Buddhist or Yogic A.A. either, although members may avail themselves of any of these, maybe more than one.

This tradition is not violated by naming your Higher Power or mentioning how a version of that Power had to be changed. No one ever objected to members trying Buddhist or Yogic meditation. The problem arises when doing any of these things becomes a requirement for membership. You need never have to be "saved" to join any A.A. group. The message must be A.A. as well, as this book sets out. Saving souls is not allowed. We save asses. We also don't do treatment. We do step work, not therapy homework. Some Dual Diagnosis groups have used materials that me be closer to therapy than carrying the message. This book does not do that.

Tradition Six

An A.A. group ought never endorse, finance or lend the A.A. name to any related facility or outside enterprise lest problems of money, property, and prestige divert us from our primary purpose.

Neither A.A. or any Dualaholic group or fellowship endorses any hospital, treatment center, recovery house or club. We also do not endorse any publishers (except A.A. World Services and the A.A. Grapevine, although if Dualaholics have an internal magazine, that is also part of us, whomever us is).

Courts are not part of A.A. We invite its participants into open meetings at first and closed meetings (where they still exist) if the person has a desire to stop drinking. Those who only used and do not identify as alcoholic cannot attend closed meetings and should not share in open ones unless the pain is too great. We urge participants to seek some other higher power than the Court. It is impossible to have a spiritual awakening based on fear. Court participants with mental illness are, of course, invited to Dualaholic meetings. Dualaholic meetings that do not want casual attendees getting their slips signed should probably vote their meetings closed and not sign slips.

Tradition Seven

Every A.A. group ought to be fully self-supporting, declining outside contributions.

Many people individualize this tradition in their own lives. Poverty is an attractive spiritual virtue that you can take on, but certainly you do not have to, and especially not at the expense of family members who are then required to help.

If a member dies, do not take money from the survivors (although a Club can). Indeed, you may need to take up a collection to help them.

The biggest issue is rent. Many clubs simply have you give them all contributions because running such a club is a precarious exercise. Don't do it. Leave some token amount every meeting so that you will have your own treasury to give to the Central Office or service committees, including the General Service Board.

Church basements present a different problem. Sometimes in trying to help you, they under-charge rent. That is fine for new groups, but as you grow, up the rent. This is even more the case if you have meetings at hospitals or government buildings. Always pay something unless you are taking a meeting to the patients, but don't let that free meeting be where your home group meets.

Lastly, don't overdo the snacks at the expense of either rent or contributions. Have someone bake or buy something, but if you are a poor group, make sure they know this is voluntary on their part.

Tradition Eight

Alcoholics Anonymous should remain forever non-professional, but our service centers may employ special workers.

Unless your therapist or doctor is fellow sufferer, they cannot be a member. While in the distant future, if we become a separate entity, we might have our General Service Office with professional advisors and liaisons. That is not today. We don't ask therapists how to vote on group matters unless something is seriously wrong nor do they get a say on the A.A. Program, the original and any modifications for Dualaholics.

Tradition Nine

A.A., as such, ought never be organized; but we may create service boards or committees directly responsible to those they serve.

These committees are where General Service Representatives go. In some places, the District meets monthly and the Area (the state or part of a state) meet quarterly. In metro areas they meet together. Every two years, areas elect a Delegate to the General Service Conference in New York City (or environs) and they advise and are assisted by the General Services Board, although the Conference is the decision-making body, their decisions are guided by input from the group GSRs. As such, it is an upside-down hierarchy with members of groups on the top, all guided by a higher power.

The General Services Office, A.A. World Services (our publishing arm) and A.A. Grapevine/La Viña (magazines) works under the General Services Board day-to-day. So far, special constituencies are not represented other than by their GSRs. This is probably a good thing, so there probably won't be a special Dualaholic Delegate.

Tradition Ten

Alcoholics Anonymous has no opinion on outside issues: hence the A.A. name ought never be drawn into public controversy.

We have no opinion on Drug Court (except our relations with them), dry and wet counties, legalization, who's elected to what office, either the sanctity or equality of marriage, the difficulty or ease of drug, alcohol or mental health commitment or who gets to shoot off the fireworks at the Fourth of July.

We will serve any alcoholics or dualaholics anywhere when needed, including prisoners, patients and deployed members of the armed forces. This non-opinion keeps us from fighting amongst ourselves in public or meetings and we have no issues committees except our services structure, which handles inside issues, mostly books and pamphlets. This lets politically-minded newcomers work on themselves and not the world while at A.A. Some members become entirely non-political and others are elected officials. We have no opinion on that either.

We are not problem free, as we struggle with making the rooms safe for everyone. While there are fellowships for people with sexual addictions, most are co-addicted to alcohol, drugs and may be Dualaholic. This problem is not going away. If anyone feels bothered, say something. Your safety is not an outside issue.

Tradition Eleven

Our public relations policy is based on attraction rather than promotion; we need always maintain personal anonymity at the level of press, radio, and films.

A.A. does run ads to help people find both national and local contact information, but we don't show our faces. If the face is clear, it's a hired actor. Real actors who are real alcoholics or dualaholics are not shown. There are no celebrity endorsements, although we can sometimes tell who's a member. If we have direct knowledge that someone is, we don't mention it, in or out of the rooms. We are generally careful when eating out together to watch how we talk, however, unless we are celebrities, media ourselves or politicians, the world does not care if we are members, so this tradition probably does not apply.

It is certainly no excuse for not making an amend to your employer. Not breaking your anonymity at work is not a thing, especially if you go to lunch meetings and then come back with carryout. Most employers will be accommodating and if they are not, you can take legal action. If you are new and your firm has an employee assistance program (EAP), using it is not a bad idea (although we don't officially endorse such things and they are not part of A.A.).

Tradition Twelve

Anonymity is the spiritual foundation of all our traditions, ever reminding us to place principles before personalities.

This is not just a redo of Tradition Eleven. This is internal anonymity. Let us say your counselor is a member. When he or she is in the rooms or speaking for you at your anniversary, he or she is just an alcoholic or dualaholic. If some celebrity walks into your meeting, especially an early evening or afternoon meeting, then it is because they need the meeting, not so you can ooh and aah over them. They are just another drunk. Say a member of the General Service Board is visiting the area and goes to your meeting? Just another drunk. We are all the same. It is how we stay sober and how we stay alive. We can't find God any other way.

www.ingramcontent.com/pod-product-compliance
Lightning Source LLC
Chambersburg PA
CBHW030512220526
45464CB00006B/2763